Look Bigger and Better

Get Big Arms Now, Sculpt A V-Shaped Torso, Look Better Instantly For Men, The Ultimate No-Weight Workout

Lee L. Boyce

Look Bigger and Better: Get Big Arms Now, Sculpt A V-Shaped Torso, Look Better Instantly For Men, The Ultimate No-Weight Workout

This book was self-published with the amazing help of <u>Self-Publishing Made Easy Now!</u> [1] . You can grab a free copy of the checklist that started my journey here: <u>FREE Self-Publishing Checklist</u> [2] .

[1] https://selfpublishingmadeeasynow.com/xpjv

[2] https://selfpublishingmadeeasynow.com/free_checklist

Table of Contents

Book 1 - Get Big Arms Now

Easy Secrets To Get Your Arms Bulging

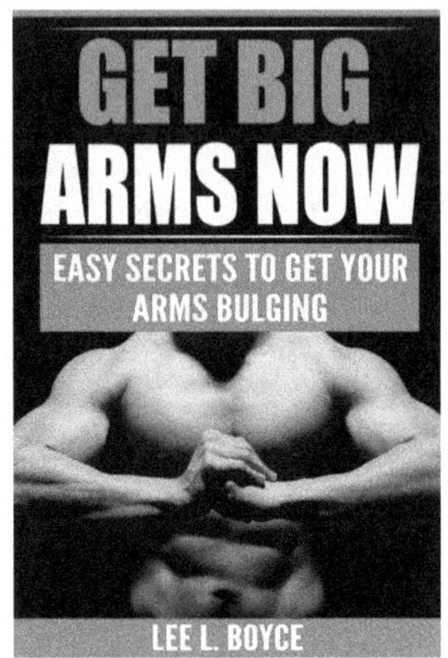

1 - Introduction

Admit it. One of the main reasons why you lift weights is because you want to build big arms and chest. That's because even with a shirt on, these muscle groups will define your physique. You don't even have to expose them like the abdominal muscles.

Just look at every movie poster with Dwayne 'The Rock' Johnson on it. It can't be overemphasized how much the size of his arms makes him look strong and intimidating. Well, you can say that genetics plays a big part in how the Jumanji star looks, and that's scientifically correct. But even when you don't have a DNA signature that spells 'tree trunk-sized arms', it's still possible to maximize the potentials of what you inherited.

Before you devote the remaining years of your life doing endless sets of dumbbell curls to get your own 'big guns', there's actually more to getting bigger arms than isolating that two-headed muscle. Even exercises like the bench press and chin up may contribute to arm growth, but more on that later.

In this eBook, you'll learn everything you need to know to

get big arms if you don't already have one yet, as well as bigger ones if you've somewhat hit a plateau.

2 - The Biceps

Everybody wants big biceps. When you are asked to flex a muscle, what do you usually do? Yes. You flex your biceps. Not your chest, back, or legs. No other muscle group signifies strength (at least superficially) like biceps do because they are the most visible. Even great bodybuilding champions work hard on their biceps to impress the judges.

There is a number of exercises that stimulate the bicep muscles, and some are better than the others. The biceps muscle is two-headed one of which is longer than the others. The best bicep exercises should be able to target both heads to provide the most stimulus possible. If you want to build muscle mass, focus on standing barbell curls, single arm preacher curls, incline dumbbell curls, and hammer curls.

Barbell Curl

The biceps curl is still the most effective and most basic exercise in growing your bicep muscles. You can also do it in more ways than one. You can stand with a dumbbell on each arm and curl both arms at the same time or alternating. In a concentration curl, you rest an arm on your inner thigh. You can use a preacher bench to isolate the bicep muscles. Bicep exercises are all about elbow flexion and the most basic and most effective of them all is the standing barbell curl.

How to Perform:

- Using a shoulder-width grip, hold a barbell with your palms facing front. The arms should be straight and pointing to the floor. Elbows should be locked around an inch from the sides. This is the starting position.

- Bending your elbows, slowly curl the barbell towards your chest while keeping your back and elbows fixed.

- When the bar reaches the front of your chest, contract the bicep muscles and hold the position for a second.

- Slowly lower down the barbell as you resist the weight until your arms are straight and you're back to the starting position. That would be one repetition.

Single Arm Dumbbell Preacher Curl

This is another great isolation exercise for your biceps. The single arm dumbbell preacher curl's stress focus is on the biceps' peak (found on the muscle's short head). This exercise adds some fullness of the biceps' lower portion, making it one of the best exercises in building arm mass.

How to Perform:

- Sit on a preacher bench and hold the dumbbell using an underhand grip. The arm should be in an extended position and almost straight. The elbow should be firmly locked. This is the starting position.

- Bending on the elbow, slowly lift the dumbbell up by curling the weight towards the shoulder. You should keep your upper arm resting on the preacher board during the entire motion.

- When the dumbbell is almost touching your shoulder, contract the bicep muscles and hold for a second.

- Slowly lower down the dumbbell while resisting the weight until the arm is almost straight and you're back to the starting position. That would be one repetition.

Incline Dumbbell Curl

If you want more mass in your biceps, you must incorporate

an exercise that stretches them. The incline dumbbell curl falls second only to the standing barbell curl as far as muscle mass building is concerned. It's because it allows full range of motion for the arms and gives that great stretch on the biceps right at the bottom of the routine. You should use less weight than you would in a barbell curl because this exercise is much more difficult. If you're thinking how this exercise can build more mass if you'll be using less resistance, the secret lies in following the strict form and that amazing pump you'll feel after a full set.

How to Perform:

- Hold a dumbbell on each arm and sit on an incline bench. Your arms should be straight and pointing to the ground. Palms should be facing your trunk. Slowly lay your back flat on the bench. This will be the starting position.

- Slowly bend on the elbows and curl both arms. As your hand approaches your chest while raising the dumbbells, turn the palms so they face you.

- When the dumbbells are almost touching your shoulder, contract the bicep muscles and hold for a second.

- Slowly lower down the dumbbells while resisting the weight until the arms are almost straight and you're back to the starting position. That would be one repetition.

You can also do alternating curls if you want, instead of lifting both arms at the same time. A complete repetition would be one you've done curling one arm and the other.

Hammer Curl

The hammer curl is not really a biceps exercise, but it targets the brachialis, the muscle at the lower end of your biceps and is the elbow's strongest flexor. The brachialis runs along the upper arm's side. Targeting the brachialis will lend a great degree of enhancement to the overall size of your biceps. When fully developed, it gives the impression of a tennis ball under your skin between the triceps and the biceps. This pushes the biceps up and creates a muscle peak, filling out the lower part of the biceps and providing thickness in the area.

How to Perform:

- Standing up, hold a dumbbell in each hand. Your arms must be straight on the sides and pointed to the ground. The palms should be facing your trunk. This will be the starting position.

- Bending on the elbow, slowly lift the dumbbells up by curling the weight towards the shoulder. You must keep your palms facing your trunk throughout the exercise and you should feel the burn on your forearms and the brachialis muscle.

- When the dumbbells are almost touching your shoulder, contract the bicep muscles and hold for a second.

- Slowly lower down the dumbbells while resisting the weight until the arms are almost straight and you are back to the starting position. That would be one repetition.

You can also do alternating hammer curls if you want, instead of lifting both arms at the same time. One repetition would be one you've done curling one arm and the other.

3 - Triceps

Triceps are often referred to as the unsung heroes of big arms. Most people think that building big biceps is enough. What they don't realize is that the triceps comprise more than two-thirds of the upper arm muscles. Imagine what the overall size will be if these muscles are properly developed.

While the bicep muscles are stimulated using curling or pulling movements, the triceps, being on the other side of the upper arm can be targeted using pushing movements. You need your biceps to work on your back muscles while you need your triceps to work on your chest and muscle shoulders.

Because triceps are larger and stronger than biceps, you need a bit more effort to stimulate them to grow. You'll need to incorporate exercises that work on the triceps in multiple angles. The best triceps exercises include the dips, close grip bench presses, triceps pushdowns, skull crushers, and extensions.

Dips

The dip is one of the best triceps exercises mainly because you don't even need any specialized equipment to perform it. You can simply use a chair or two benches. However, the dip exercise is best performed on parallel bars, which you can find in most gyms. You can change the resistance or weight by using more of your body weight during the routine. When you get stronger, you can start adding more weight belts or putting extra weight plates on your lap.

How to Perform:

- Hoist your body up on the parallel bars. Your arms should be straight and elbows should be locked. The torso should be perpendicular to the floor, and your feet should not be touching the ground. The knees should be slightly bent and the ankles should be crossed. Maintain this torso and leg posture through-out the routine. This will be the starting position.

- Slowly bend on the elbows as you lower your body towards the ground. Do this until the shoulder joints are just below the elbows.

- Push your body up slowly until the elbows are almost straight and you're back to the starting position. That would be one repetition.

Close Grip Bench Presses

The bench press is the best exercise for the chest and the core, but if you change the grip a bit, you can also use it to build bigger triceps. While the standard bench press starts with a wider than a shoulder-width grip, placing the hands nearer each other makes the triceps work harder as the movement becomes less dependent on the chest muscles. And when you develop stronger triceps, your bench press improves, too.

How to Perform:

- Lay down with your back flat on a bench. Using an overhand grip, grasp the barbell. Your hands should be apart by a shoulder width, and your arms should be straight and pointing up. This will be the starting position.

- Slowly lower down the bar straight until it almost touches your chest. Pause for one second.

- Slowly press the bar up by pushing with your arms until they are straight and you're back to the starting position. That would be one repetition.

Tricep Pushdowns

The tricep pushdown is considered by many as the best tricep exercise. If you haven't included it in your own routine, you're definitely missing out on its benefits. The tricep pushdown isolates and targets your triceps, but only if you do it with proper form. Using more weight than what is necessary will involve the shoulder and back muscles, which defeats the purpose. The trick here is to imagine that you have a rope wrapped around your shoulders and upper arms, keeping them down. If this is a bit difficult for you, you're most likely using too much weight.

How to Perform:

- Grab on the short bar or the rope handle attached to a cable station's high pulley. Pull on the cable until your upper arms are tucked in your sides. You should do an overhand grip with your hands a shoulder-width apart. This will be your starting position.

- Slowly push down on the bar or pull the rope handle until your elbows are locked in a straight position. Pause for a second.

- Slowly bend on the elbows until you're back to the

starting position. You should keep your upper arms tucked into the side throughout the exercise. That would be one repetition.

Skull Crushers

The skull crushers, also known as French presses or Lying Tricep Extensions, got their moniker because you need to lower down the barbell until the bar almost touches your forehead as if crushing your skull. It's another great tricep isolation exercise, and doing high reps gives a great pump of blood into your triceps. This pump is essential in speeding up muscle growth, as well as promoting muscle repair.

How to Perform:

- Lay flat on your back on a bench. Have someone hand you a barbell or a couple of dumbbells. This is a difficult exercise so don't use too much weight. Your arms should be a shoulder-width apart, straight, and locked. You should use an overhand grip with your arms pointing up. This will be the starting position.

- Slowly bend on the elbows while keeping the upper arms perpendicular to the ground and until the bar almost touches the forehead. Pause for a second.

- Slowly lift the barbell up by straightening up your arms and you're back to the starting position. That would be one repetition.

Overhead Extensions

If you want bigger muscles, you must attack them at every angle possible to stimulate the most amount of muscle fibers possible. This is what the overhead extension does. It's the only real stretch-position exercise for your triceps. You can use a barbell, dumbbells, or a cable system. You can do both arms at the same time or alternate them. The overhead extensions work on the long head of the triceps.

How to Perform:

- Grab a dumbbell and sit on a bench. Lift the dumbbell over your head and grip the top end with both hands while forming a diamond shape. Your upper arms should be perpendicular to the ground and the elbows are slightly bent. This would be the starting position.

- Slowly lower down the dumbbell by bending on the elbow. Keep your chest strong and your shoulders still throughout the movement.

- Slowly raise the dumbbell by pushing with your triceps until you are back to the starting position. That would be one repetition.

4 - Forearms

What good are big biceps and triceps if the forearms are left out? Although you might already be working out your forearms while doing all the exercises for your upper arms, there are specific exercises you can include in your routine to help build them.

Stimulating forearm growth is a bit difficult since it's always almost used when you use your arms. They are tough and resilient to growth so you need to consider intensity and varying angles of stimulation.

Wrist Curl

This is the best isolation exercise for your forearm, but unfortunately, it is often ignored by many. The movement targets your forearm without employing other muscles like the biceps during hammer curls. The wrist curl is just like the bicep curl but instead of bending on your elbows, you bend on your wrist.

How to Perform:

- Grab a dumbbell and sit on a bench. Put the lower arm holding the dumbbell on your thigh. The hand should hang over the knee and the palm should be facing up. This will be the starting position.

- Slowly lower down the dumbbell by hyperextending at the wrist.

- Slowly lift up the dumbbell by curling at the wrist. You should feel the burn on your forearm muscle. That would be one repetition.

Reverse Wrist Curl

This exercise works out the other side of your forearm for that 360-degree workout on your lower arms. This is pretty much the same as a wrist curl but you start with the palms facing down.

Reverse Barbell Curl

This exercise also works out your biceps because you are curling on the elbows, but it stimulates the brachialis as well as the forearms. You should use less weight than you would on a standard barbell curl.

How to Perform:

- Using a shoulder-width grip, hold a barbell with an

overhand grip. The arms should be straight and pointing to the floor. Elbows should be locked around an inch from the sides. This is the starting position.

- Bending on your elbows, slowly curl the barbell towards your chest while keeping your back and elbows fixed. Pause for a second.

- Slowly lower down the barbell as you resist the weight until your arms are straight and you're back to the starting position. That would be one repetition.

5 - Arm Training Tips from the Experts

Don't Overtrain

Your arms are used in your daily routine and are also engaged when you're doing chest and back exercises; overtraining them is not a good idea. Limit hitting a muscle group to two times a week, maximum.

Size First, Shape Later

Don't go drooling over those big arms featured in magazines. You might not have the genetic makeup for it. What you can do, however, is to maximize their growth potential. Focus on building mass first by doing heavy weights with lower reps. The shape will follow eventually.

Train the Supporting Muscles

Doing other exercises that might not seem to be working your arms can do wonders in building more muscle mass on both the biceps and the triceps. Basically, when you work out the chest muscles and the shoulders, you also engage the triceps, and when you do your back exercises like pull-ups and rows, you also work on your biceps.

Follow Proper Form

This tip goes out to all exercise routines. Form is more important than the amount of resistance involved. Proper form helps prevent injuries and it ensures that only the targeted muscles are stimulated, allowing for better and faster growth and recovery.

Warm Up

This can't be reiterated enough. Your muscles should first be conditioned and warmed up before you can use them at their full potential. Make sure to do light cardio and stretching before you take on your strength training program.

6 - Conclusion

Big arms are a combination of properly developed and trained biceps, triceps, and forearms. Leaving out one just doesn't cut it. The trick is to aim for proper form, intensity, and just enough weight to stimulate growth, but not too much that you engage other muscle groups.

Book 2 - Sculpt A V-Shaped Torso

Perfect Tricks and Tips For Sculpting

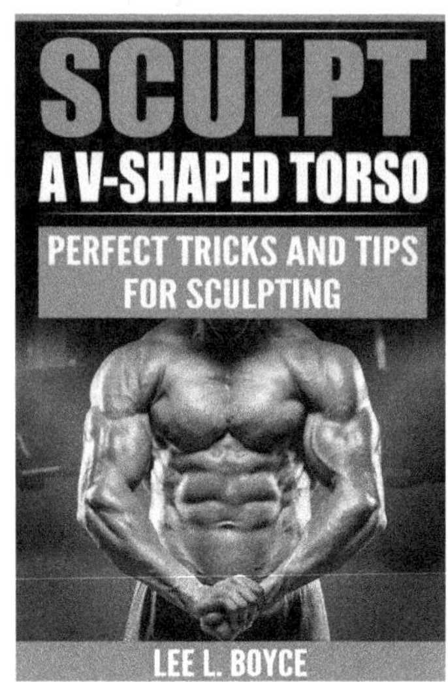

1 - Introduction

Bodybuilding has existed for the longest time. While different people have different views of what they believe is the ideal body shape, one of the classic forms bodybuilders covet is a V-shaped torso. A thick back with broad shoulders that taper down into a trim waist creates the V-shape that a lot of people find attractive. Having a torso shaped like this is very masculine, regardless of one's overall body mass. While this body form is very ideal for men, a V-shaped torso also looks very nice for women.

Achieving this body form takes a lot of work. You might have tried and failed to achieve a chiseled upper body, but you can now get it with the help of this book. We will teach you the right approach for getting a torso of mythical proportions. From developing the right muscle groups to building thick and ripped muscles, this is your ultimate guide to proper upper body sculpting. If you are ready to sculpt your upper body to resemble that of superheroes, this guide will show you the way.

2 - Components of a V-Shaped Torso

Molding your upper body takes a holistic approach to body-building. You will need to work on multiple groups of muscles to create that V-shaped torso. You will need to work on 3 regions of your upper body to shape your torso to a V. These regions are your back, your shoulders, and your abdomen.

Each of these 3 regions plays a role in creating that V-shaped torso you've always dreamed of. Beyond molding your body to the shape that you want, working on the muscles in these regions can enhance your overall physical performance.

1. Back

Building a big, strong back is the first step in sculpting an imposing upper body. Working on your back muscles, especially the lats, will help you accomplish exactly that. Beyond creating the broad base of your V torso, a sturdy back will also greatly improve your overall body strength.

There are 2 approaches to building your back muscles for

attaining that V shape: adding width and adding thickness. Different exercises will help in building wide and thick back muscles. You cannot sculpt an imposing back musculature without accomplishing both of these.

2. Shoulders

The second essential component of a V-shaped torso are the shoulders. Having thick, broad shoulders greatly enhances the V shape of your upper body. When combined with a toned back, bulked-up shoulders will make the upper part of your torso stand out, with or without clothes on. The main muscle you have to work on this region is the deltoids. Having thick, well-rounded deltoids will help create very imposing shoulders, perfect for that V-shaped torso you are aiming to build.

3. Abdomen

As part of your core, the abdomen is a critical area to work on for any fitness junkie. Toned abs will greatly enhance the center of gravity of your body, improving strength, flexibility, and balance. Just as important, toned abs look very attractive, regardless of what body type you have. Slimming and toning your abdominal muscles is the final and perhaps the most difficult step in building a V-shaped torso. The rectus abdominis muscle is the main muscle you should work on here.

3 - Back Exercises

The back is composed of multiple muscles, with the most important one being the latissimus dorsi, better known as the lats. Bodybuilders of all levels will benefit from working on their back, as it improves both your physical form and your performance.

For those who want to get a V-shaped torso, working on your back is a must. You should work on both the width and thickness of your back muscles to sculpt your upper body. Here are some of the exercises that are highly recommended for strengthening and sculpting your back.

1. Deadlift

The deadlift is a classic exercise that any bodybuilder can't miss out on. More than just an exercise that strengthens your back, the deadlift will also build your calves, traps, and buttocks. Aside from working on a wide range of muscles, regularly performing this exercise help release muscle-building hormones, strengthen your bone structure, and help you get big and strong right away.

The deadlift is best done during the start of your workout, as you can lift high amounts of weight while warming up muscles all over your body. With the weight (use a barbell) on the floor, bend your knees to grab the bar, and pull the bar to the middle of your thighs while locking your hips and knees. Return the weight to the floor by moving your hips back and bending your legs. Keep your back neutral at all times while doing deadlifts, as rounding or arching it can cause serious injury.

2. Pull-ups

The pull-up is one of the most popular bodyweight exercises of all time. Considered as one of the essential exercises for bulking up your back, this also works on your arms, shoulders, and abs. The pull-up is a superb compound exercise that will test and build your upper body strength. All you need is a bar that can support your body weight and you can get started right away.

The steps to doing the proper pull-up are simple. Grip the bar with your hands about shoulder-width apart. Get your feet off the floor by bending your knees and straightening your arms. While keeping your midsection contracted by tightening your abs, pull yourself up by pulling your elbows down to the floor. Go all the way up until your chin passes the bar. Go back to starting position by lowering yourself slowly until your arms are straight. Perform as many reps as you can.

3. Bent-over rows

You can use either a barbell or a pair of dumbbells to perform a bent-over row. This exercise mainly targets the muscles of your middle back, but it also triggers the other back muscles as well as the shoulders. You can also use a great amount of weight with this exercise, which is helpful for developing overall strength and muscle mass.

Hold the barbell with a pronated grip. If you are using a pair of dumbbells, hold them shoulder-width apart. Slightly bend your knees and straighten your back, bending your torso until it is almost parallel to the floor. While keeping your torso stationary, pull the weight towards you by squeezing your back muscles. Slowly return the weight to starting position. Do about 6 to 10 reps per set, only using the amount of weight that your body can tolerate.

4. Seated cable rows

Just like the bent-over row, the seated cable row mainly works on your middle back and shoulders. To perform this exercise, you'll need a low pulley rowing machine that has a

V-bar. You can also use a straight bar, performing this exercise with a pronated grip. You can work on different muscles of your back by modifying the width of your grip and flipping your grip.

Sit on the machine, with your feet firmly planted on the front platform with your knees slightly bent, and firmly grip the V-bar or straight bar using your desired grip and width. With your arms straight, lean over while keeping your natural back alignment until your back forms a 90-degree angle with your thighs. Pull back the handles toward your torso by squeezing your back until it touches your abdomen. Slowly go back to starting position. Avoid swinging your torso to avoid back injury.

5. Lat pull-down

The lat pull-down is a great exercise that targets the upper back. Aside from working on your lats, this exercise is also great in building your lower back and core.

Sit at the lat pull-down station of your exercise machine, sitting directly underneath the bar. Grip the bar with an overhand grip with your hands a shoulder-width apart. In starting position, your arms should be completely straight up and your torso at an upright position. Pull the bar all the way to your collarbone by pulling your shoulder blades down and back. Slowly return to your starting position to complete 1 rep. Make sure to keep your back neutral at all times.

4 - Shoulder Exercises

Bulking up your shoulders is one of the ways to create a more defined upper body. Broad, well-rounded shoulders will work with any kind of body, but they stand out best when combined with a chiseled torso. Building your shoulder muscles, most especially the deltoids, will make your upper body broader and create a more dramatic V-taper that will turn heads.

Building all 3 heads of the deltoids is crucial to make your shoulders stand out from all angles. This list of exercises will help you get those cannonball shoulders that have both mass and definition.

1. Shoulder press

The shoulder press, also known as the military press, is the ultimate shoulder exercise. Working on all 3 heads of the deltoids, while also involving the arms, traps, and chest, the shoulder press is an exercise that challenges your upper body strength. You can use the barbell for a more full-body workout or a shoulder press machine to better isolate your shoulder muscles.

To perform a shoulder press using a barbell, lift the bar using a pronated grip and place it at the level of your shoulders (or you can use the help of a spotter). The ideal grip length is slightly wider than shoulder width. The standing position of this exercise is a highly challenging full-body workout, while the seated version spares your lower back a little bit. Lift the bar up over your head by locking your arms, holding it at shoulder level. Lower the bar to starting position to complete 1 rep. Do about 8 to 12 reps per set.

2. Front raise

The front raise is a shoulder exercise that mainly targets the front head of your deltoids. Performing this exercise together with your usual shoulder routine will build up the front portion of your shoulders. You can perform this exercise using a barbell, dumbbells, cables, or resistance bands as your source of resistance.

Get into starting position by standing with your feet a shoulder-width apart from each other. With your elbows slightly bent, hold your choice or resistance with both hands. Lift your arm up until your arms are up over your head, keeping your elbows slightly bent throughout. Return to starting position to complete one rep. Do about 8 to 12 reps per set or until fatigue sets in.

3. Lateral raises

This exercise is basically the same as the front raise. This time, you will lift your arms to the sides. This exercise will specifically attack the lateral head of your deltoids, working up the sides of your shoulder in the process. While you can use different sources of resistance for this exercise, this is best done using a pair of dumbbells with a weight that puts the most resistance on your shoulders.

Pick the dumbbells up and place them on the sides. With your elbows slightly bent and your torso at a neutral position, lift the dumbbells until at least level with your shoulders. Your hands should be slightly tilted forward like when you're pouring water in a glass. Pause for a second, then slowly bring down the weight to the starting position. Do about 8 to 12 reps per set or until fatigue sets in.

4. Bent-over raises

This exercise mainly targets the muscles located at the rear part of your shoulders, most especially the rear head of your deltoids. While this exercise can be performed while standing, the bent-over raise is best recommended while sitting down to reduce the stress placed in the back.

To get into starting position, sit at the edge of the bench with your feet together and dumbbells on hand placed just behind your legs. Bend your waist while keeping your back straight until it forms a 45-degree angle with the floor. Lift the dumbbells straight to the side until both of your arms are parallel to the floor. Slowly lower the dumbbells to starting position. Do about 8 to 12 reps per set or until fatigue sets in.

5 - Abdominal Exercises

A massive back and broad shoulders set the tone for creating a V-shaped torso. A trimmed midsection will complete it. Beyond getting a trim abdomen, it pays to have a ripped one. This is where working on your abdomen comes into the picture. Strengthening one's core is a must for any hardcore bodybuilder, and a trim midsection will always attract stares.

It must be noted that the exercises mentioned here mainly focus on building the abs (the six-pack), as excessively building your obliques (the muscles at the sides of your abdomen) may widen your midsection.

1. Crunches

The crunch is the most basic abs exercise. It has more than enough variations to work on all regions of your abdomen and to keep you challenged. While some would say that this exercise is an ineffective means for slimming and toning your waist, it is actually an exercise that provides results if done the right way.

To do crunches, lay flat on your back with your knees bent and feet hip-length apart. Place your hand behind your head, but don't make your hands support the weight of your head. With your back staying straight, lift up your torso by contracting your abdominal muscles. Without relaxing your abs, go back to starting position to complete one rep. When doing crunches, it is important to never yank your neck or back, do not use your body's momentum to lift your body, and do not hold your breath.

2. Planks

The plank is another bodyweight exercise that not just emphasizes your abs but also works on all the muscles of your midsection. The plank is ideal for building overall core strength. There are also multiple variations of the plank available, but even the basic version of it is more than enough to give you that much-needed abdominal workout.

To perform the plank, get your body in the push-up position, bend your elbows at a 90-degree angle, and let your body weight rest on your forearms. Form a straight line using your body, contracting your midsection to hold that position. Hold this position for 30 seconds or for as long as you can. To increase the intensity of this exercise, you can increase the time you hold this position.

3. Seated leg pull-in

The seated leg pull-in applies tension squarely to your rectus abdominis muscle, while also working on your hip flexors. The lower portion of your abs will benefit the most from this exercise. Given that traditional abdominal exercises such as sit-ups target the upper/middle region of your abs, this is a must-include in your workout list.

Sit on the edge of the bench with your legs stretched out in front of you, feet together. Lean your torso to a 45-degree angle with the bench, using your arms to support the weight of your body. To perform one rep, bring your knees towards your torso while you pull your torso upward, keeping your midsection contracted and your back stable at all times. Go back to starting position to complete 1 rep.

4. Leg raises

The leg raise is another exercise that will target the lower part of your abs. Just like the crunches, this is a simple and highly-effective way for toning up your midsection. This is another exercise that is a must include in your workout routine if you aim to get a V-shaped torso.

To perform this exercise, lie flat on the floor or a flat bench with your legs together. While keeping your legs straight and together, lift it all the way up until your butt is off the floor. Lower your legs, stopping just before they hit the floor, to complete one rep.

6 - Must-Know Stuff to Build Your Dream Body

Exercise is a critical part of building a V-shaped torso. However, you might have some habits that could be preventing you from achieving your dream body. Building a V-shaped torso goes beyond putting the work in the gym. You will also have to work on things such as nutrition and rest.

At the same time, there are some workout habits that you should develop to get the best results at all times. Here is a collection of tips that will help you not just get a V-shaped torso, but will also help you get into the best shape of your life.

1. Follow a balanced diet

Being physically fit goes beyond following a strict workout routine. The way you eat also plays a huge factor in helping (or hindering) you achieve your fitness goals, may it be achieving a V-taper or completing a marathon.

Put an emphasis on eating fresh food, as they are loaded with more nutrients without an excess of calories, salt, and preservatives. Make sure to get enough protein to build up your muscles, carbohydrates, and fat to keep your energy sources replenished, and vitamins and minerals to keep your bodily functions working.

2. Get enough rest

Rest is a completely underrated part of the muscle-building process. It is during rest when your body recuperates and your muscles get their much-needed chance to heal from both fatigue and injuries. While you are resting, your body builds up muscle mass.

So if you are working hard in the gym and you're still not getting enough results, you might be working out too much. Properly spacing your workouts and adding rest days will help you achieve better results. Also, make sure to get enough sleep on a daily basis.

3. Follow proper form when training

Form is a very important component of training. Practicing proper form and technique is important in exercising because it ensures that all involved muscles are properly stimulated. Also, following proper form is crucial for preventing injuries, especially if you are dealing with heavy weights.

To ensure that you are following proper form, review your technique. Read up on the proper execution of exercises and evaluate if you are doing it right. You can also ask the help of a spotter, trainer, or someone more experienced than you to evaluate and improve your form.

7 - Conclusion

You have just read a simplified guide on how you can get a V-shaped torso. By following these exercises, improving your habits, and staying disciplined, you can get that ripped and tapered upper body that will turn everyone's heads.

There are more ways to get that V-taper and improve your body. By continuing with your fitness journey, learning new techniques, and pushing your body to its limits, you can achieve fitness and health that go beyond form. Good luck!

Book 3 - Look Better Instantly For Men

Amazing Tricks To Improve Your Appearance Immediately

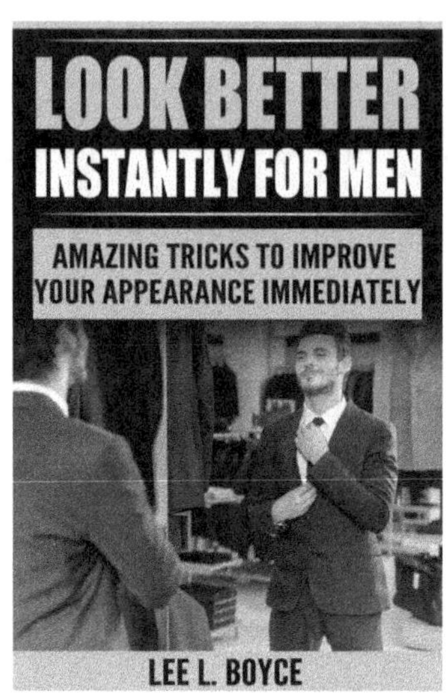

1 - Introduction

Here's the hard truth. Everyone cares about the way they look. You may not be as vain as the men you see in magazines, but whether you admit it or not, you know deep inside that looks matter, and they matter a lot if you want to make a mark in this world.

According to a study conducted by Daniel Hamermesh, people with below-average looks earn a lower salary (up to 9% less) compared to people who have average looks, while people with above-average looks earn a pay premium of almost 5% more than the people who have average looks. It may seem disheartening to some but think about it.

Is it really a surprise that attractive people are earning more money than their less-attractive counterparts? While the study may seem like it's promoting superficial standards, it's part of human nature to prefer what's pleasing to the eye. When you see something you like, you can't help but want to be close to.

So, if we're just going to base it on this study, physically attractive men seem to have it easy in life. Not only are they getting paid more, but they also have first dibs on promotions. And let's face it, they probably also have better luck with the ladies.

So, is there hope for the average Joe? Yes, there is. Fortunately, attractiveness is relative, so even if you were born with average looks, you can make yourself seem more attractive to other people, with the right tricks up your sleeve.

There is no set formula for attractiveness, rather there are many factors that come into play. But if you're going to really think about what makes people attractive, it's really just putting a bit more effort into improving your appearance and changing the way you feel about yourself.

In other words, it's developing your confidence that will instantly improve your appearance.

In this book, we'll talk about the many ways you can boost your confidence. From getting the right haircut for your face shape, to dressing for success, you'll learn the secret to becoming the man you've always wanted to be.

I wish you the best of luck!

2 - Finding the Right Hairstyle

One of the easiest ways to improve your looks is to get a haircut. Your choice of haircut doesn't just show off your personality, but it can also be a reflection of your outlook on life. This is why, if you want to make a good impression with the people that you meet, you need to make sure that your hairstyle not only suits your face shape, it also fits the image that you want to show off to the world.

But how do you know which hairstyle is right for you? Let's begin by looking at your face shape. Knowing the exact shape of your face may not seem like a big deal, but it can help you choose a more flattering haircut for yourself, as well as glasses and specs that will make you look like a million bucks.

To know what your face shape is, you need to take a good hard look in the mirror, and then, using a tape measure, measure your forehead, your cheekbones, jaw line, and face length. Once you've taken these measurements, note the part that is the most prominent of them all.

If your face length is greater than the width in between your cheekbones, and your forehead is greater than your jaw line, then you have an oval face shape. An oval face shape has a rounded jaw and looks best with a classic short cut with a side-swept parting. Avoid the forward fringe as this can increase the rounded look of the face. The ideal hairstyle for the oval face should have a volume on top to show off your facial features.

If all your measurements are evenly proportionate and you have a strong, sharp jaw line, then you have a square face shape. A square face shape is versatile enough to pull off most hairstyles, from buzz cuts to long layers, and everything in between. But take note, the shorter your haircut, the more masculine your face will look. The best haircut for the square face shape is classic and neat. Think short layers with a side parting.

If your face length is the most prominent measurement of them all, with the forehead, cheekbones, and jaw line all similar in size, then you have a rectangle face shape. A rectangular face shape is like the longer square face shape so you need to choose a hairstyle that won't elongate your face. Styles that look best on the rectangle face shape that those that allow hair to fall across the forehead and to the sides. This is a great way to add width to the face shape so that it doesn't look narrow.

If your face length and cheekbones have similar measurements and are larger than your forehead and jaw line, then you have a round face shape. A round face has a rounded chin and lacks natural angles, so you need to choose a haircut that will give it some definition.

A good style for a round face should have height on top with a sharp edge at the sides. A pompadour works well for the round face as it adds structure to the overall look. The goal is to sharpen up the soft edges of this face shape so a flat top or a front fringe also make great choices for round faces.

If your face length is the largest measurement, and you have a narrow chin and forehead, then you have a diamond face shape. Known as one of the rarer face shapes, the diamond face looks best with hairstyles that give an illusion of a wider forehead. Fringes add texture to the forehead and soften the natural angles of the diamond face shape. Try doing a side sweep to make the face look wider in the forehead area. Avoid hairstyles that are too short at the sides if you don't want your ears to look bigger than they really are.

If your forehead is wider than your cheekbones and jaw line and you have a pointed chin, then you have a heart face shape. Unlike the diamond-shaped face, the heart-shaped face looks best with hairstyles that make the forehead less prominent. Choose hairstyles with a mid-length sweep that are cut thin and light to soften the strong forehead of the heart face. Avoid tight haircuts that accentuate the heart shape's narrow chin.

If your jaw line is the largest measurement, and you have a narrow forehead, then you have a triangle face shape. A triangle face calls for the opposite treatment of the heart shape so here, volume is king. Choose hairstyles that are longer and cut with fuller sides. You want to add depth to your triangular face shape so hairstyles that bring attention to your forehead works best.

If this is all a little too much for you to handle on your own, make sure to check in with your local barber. Your barber can suggest styles that suit your face shape, and even give you styling tips so that you will always look your best.

3 - Improving Grooming and Skin Care

Whether you want to admit it or not, the way you look can have a direct effect on your self-esteem. When you take care of yourself through proper grooming and the right skin care routine, you'll look more put together, which then will make you feel better about yourself. And you don't even have to put much effort into it because all you need are these basic steps.

Shave with the best razors you can afford.

If you're shaving almost every day, then you need to stop shaving with cheap razors. A quality razor can make all the difference in your skin care routine, especially if you're always finding cuts and bumps on your face after shaving. Razors that have several blades may be very popular, but you're likely to get ingrown hair and razor burn shaving with drugstore razors.

Use after-shave

If you've been shaving all these years without using a good

aftershave, you've been doing it all wrong. The right after-shave will hydrate and soothe your skin after a nice shave, so if you want great skin, this is one step you shouldn't skip. When choosing an after-shave, make sure to go for the alcohol-free type so that it doesn't dry your skin.

Wash your face with the right cleanser

Men don't often give their skin the attention it deserves. Either you're washing your face with the wrong cleanser or you're not doing it at all. If you haven't been using the right cleanser for your skin type, now is the right time to start. You want a cleanser that can give your skin a deep cleanse while packing in some serious hydration. This way, your skin will not look dry or flaky when you face the world.

Moisturize

This step is a must in any skincare routine. Moisturizing daily will help you get smooth skin that is soft to the touch. Fortunately, there are a lot of fragrance-free products that are available on the market today, so you won't have to worry about smelling "girly". You can also choose from a wide range of all-natural or organic products if you want a straightforward product that can pack in the moisture.

Always apply sunscreen

Last but not the least, always make sure to apply sunscreen, even if you're mostly staying indoors. Pick a body moisturizer with an SPF of 30 or higher if you want to hit two birds with one stone. Applying sunscreen daily will not only decrease your risk of getting skin cancer, it will also slow down skin aging caused by excessive sun exposure.

If you're constantly under a lot of stress especially, the more that you should start putting effort into your grooming and skincare routine. Maintaining a routine may require a bit of work now but you'll be enjoying the results years down the road.

4 - Dressing with Style

Even if you don't consider yourself as naturally stylish, knowing how to dress well is a skill that every man needs to have. A style is something that you can use to stand out, but if you're working in an industry that will judge you based on how you look, style then becomes a priority.

Part of looking your best is making sure that you wear clothes that are not only appropriate to the occasion but also represent the better version of yourself. Here are some basic style tips that will help you dress well every single day.

Get the right fit

One of the easiest ways to quickly improve how you dress is to always make sure to get the right fit. Wearing ill-fitting clothes will not only make you look sloppy but also shorter or fatter than you actually are. Men often wear clothes that are a little too big for them because they feel comfortable in them or they just don't know how clothes should fit in the first place.

The only way that you'll be able to get clothes that fit is to try them on before buying them and see if it makes you look good. Spending a few extra minutes at the store to do this is absolutely worth it.

Turn to the classics

If you're still trying to develop your personal style, the classics is always the best place to start. Before you dabble into trends, you should first fill your closet with essential pieces that never go out of style.

A couple of white shirts, a pair of straight-leg jeans, some button-down shirts, a pair of chino trousers, and a crew neck jumper in a neutral color are must-haves in every man's wardrobe. You should also have tailored suit that fits you perfectly for those very special occasions.

Simple is best

People will judge you based on your style (or your lack of it) so if you want to be taken seriously, make sure to heed to this timeless piece of advice. Simple is always best. While prints may look good in certain ensembles, that doesn't mean that you should start a graphic tees collection.

Wearing a shirt or a sweater with large prints or logos make you look like you're still in college, or worse, you're off to a UFC fight. Choosing simple solid colors over wild prints is going to make people take you more seriously.

Buy the best quality for what you can afford

If you have the money, by all means, go crazy! But if you have a budget that you need to stick to, make sure to buy the best quality clothes that you can afford. Fashion is where quality should always trump quantity so before you buy a piece of clothing, try to decide if it's something that you'll be able to get maximum use out of. Just because you like something now and can afford it, doesn't mean that you should buy it.

Find your style

Once you get the hang of dressing yourself and being happy with the person that you've become, that's when you can start exploring your personal style. The key is to be confident about who you are and let that confidence grow as you try new styles. You only have to start with just one killer outfit and work your way from there.

Dressing well is actually easier than most men make it. With the right attitude and these basic style guidelines, you'll be dressing for success in no time. But don't just go in style, keep in mind that to look good you must also feel good about your self by taking care of your body.

5 - Being Confident with Your Body Language

Picture yourself at a job interview for a job that you've always wanted, or approaching an attractive woman at a bar. What do you think your body language would say about you? If you were to judge yourself from an outsider's perspective, what kind of image do you think you're projecting to other people? Are you confident and attractive? Or are you unsure and awkward?

Most people's instinct is to judge someone based on their body language. You may not be aware of it, but how you walk, talk, stand, and even laugh, can say a lot about you.

Confidence can take you places and your body language tells other people that you're someone worth knowing. If you want to know how to instantly become more attractive through body language, here are a few tips to help you out.

Maintain eye contact

Maintaining eye contact is one of the trickiest, yet simplest ways to show confidence. When you're talking with people, it often feels more natural to lower your head and look down, but that kind of body language is only telling people that you're not interested to interact with them.

If you want to make a good impression, make sure to keep your eyes forward and maintain eye contact with the person you're talking to.

Stand straight and keep your shoulders back

Another way to show that you're confident is to have proper posture. By standing straight with your shoulders back, you'll look like you are someone who knows exactly what you're doing. It may take a bit of getting used to, especially if you've been slouching all your life, but once you get used to standing straight, you'll look and feel like a new person. Try practicing in front of a full-length mirror until you see something that you like.

Walk with confidence

A confident man is an attractive man so if you're not getting second looks from people whenever you step into a room, then you need to work on your walk. If you're always rushing or sneaking, and people are always commenting on the way you enter a room, you need to practice taking slow wide steps.

By walking confidently, you're sending the message that you take pride in what you do, and you know exactly where you're going. Be the man that people naturally look to whenever you pass by.

Give firm handshakes

If there's one thing that men need to know how to do properly, it's how to give a firm handshake. There's nothing worse than reaching out for another man's hand during an introduction and feeling your hand go limp in theirs.

When you do a handshake, make sure to reach out for the other person's hand with a firm grip, give it a couple of shakes, then let go. Remember to not get carried away though. Try not to grip too hard or linger too long.

Smile

Lastly, don't forget to smile. Men who smile don't just look happier, but they also seem healthier and full of life. Smiling can make you look more approachable, and in many ways, more attractive to the people around you. When you smile, you exude a glow around you that make people want to spend more time with you.

Rather than looking happy or cheerful, try to practice giving genuine smiles to people. Genuine smiles are those that come from the eyes and not just the mouth.

By improving your body language, you're communicating to people that you're a force to be reckoned with. And while most body language happens without you even noticing, it's important to remember that action will always speak louder than words. It's only a matter of weeks before you start to notice people will treat you differently according to your body language.

6 - Conclusion

If you like the person you are, the world will take notice.

The only way that you'll learn to like yourself is by working on becoming the best person you can ever be.

I hope this book helps you realize your potential. When you care enough about your appearance, people will naturally take notice of you. They will want to work with you, learn from you, and just be around you more.

First impressions matter and if you make the effort, this could mean bigger better business and career prospects for you in the near future.

Book 4 - The Ultimate No-Weight Workout

Finally, A Solution For A Great Workout Without The Weights

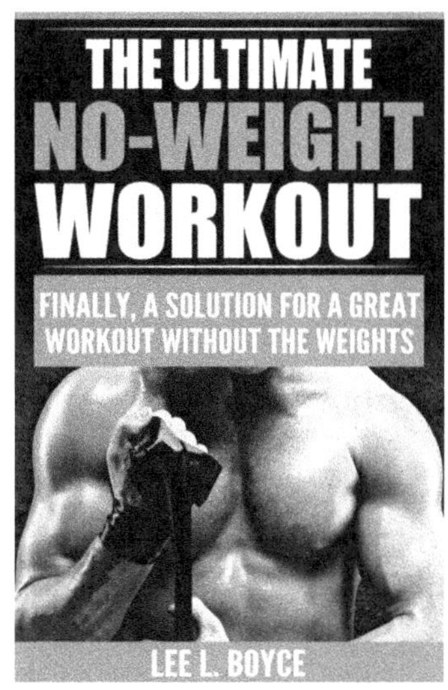

1 - Introduction

No weights? No problem.

One of the most common alibis for people who miss working out is that they don't have time to hit the gym or they don't want to spend money on exercise equipment and free weights. Although exercise aids can enhance the experience, they're really not that necessary for someone to have a good full body workout at home or any place desired.

This ebook will show you how you can get that full body strength training without the use of specialized exercise equipment, specifically free weights. You'll be working the upper body muscles which include the chest, back, shoulders, and arms and also the lower body like your thighs, buttocks, and calves. And all of these without using free weights.

Whether your goal is to build a bit of muscle, lose those extra pounds or just simply tone up, these exercises will help you reach your goal.

2 - The Chest

The bench press is still the best exercise in building chest muscles. But using this routine, you'll be toning up those pectorals all in the comfort of your own home. The best workout for your chest, without using weights, is the good old pushup. You might say it's not challenging but you'll change your mind after going through these exercises.

Standard pushup

Begin by lying face down on the floor and your hands directly under the shoulders. Keep your back straight so that the shoulders and the feet form a rigid, straight line.

Pushing with your arms, slowly and steadily lift the torso while keeping the back and legs straight and rigid. Keep doing this until the arms are straight, then slowly lower down the body by bending your arms until they form a 90-degree angle. That would be one repetition.

For beginners, you may start by putting your knees on the floor while doing the standard pushup. This reduces the body weight that you should lift up.

The standard pushup works out the whole chest and should

be the first pushup routine you should be familiar with before moving on to more advanced variations.

Incline pushup

This is similar to the standard pushup, but you need to elevate the upper body using a chair, desk, or bench. Make sure that the furniture doesn't move to avoid injuries.

Lying face down with the hands on the chair and positioned a little wider than shoulder-width. Your feet should also be a hip-width apart and your toes on the floor.

Do the same motion as the standard pushup but when going down, your chest should be just a few inches from the chair. The incline pushup works out your lower and side chest muscles. This is also an easier variation of the pushup because when you are inclined, you use less body weight for resistance.

Elevated pushup

Use the same chair or bench you used in the inclined pushup. Get on the floor using the standard pushup position but this time, place your feet on the chair instead of the ground. You should use a sturdy chair that can support your weight. For added stability, place the chair against the wall.

Do the same motion as you would with the standard pushup. You'll find this a bit more challenging because you'll be pushing more body weight than compared to doing the standard or the inclined pushup.

The elevated pushup works out your upper chest muscles and shoulders.

Advanced pushup variations

The gorilla pushup – Do a basic pushup but do it rapidly so you launch your upper body off the ground, and then clap or slap your chest before returning the hands to the starting position.

Wide pushup – You can widen the position of your hands when doing a standard pushup. This will engage more of the side chest muscles.

Narrow pushup – Position your hands nearer together while doing the pushup motion. This exercise engages more of the inner chest muscles.

3 - The Back

This is the biggest muscle group in your body and having strong back muscles can make a lot of physical work easier. They're also great to have when you need to wear that tank top or that muscle shirt on the beach. Again, if you want really huge back muscles, you should consider using free weights. But if your goal is just to tone up your core back muscles, these exercises are all you need.

Hip Hinge

The hip hinge is the most basic exercise you can do to tone up your back muscles. You simply crease at your hips and flex your torso forward then go back to straight, standing position. But even a simple exercise like the hip hinge can be ruined by poor execution.

You should check for alignment before you begin the exercise. This is best done with a mirror. The ankles, hips, shoulders, and ears should be vertically aligned. This would be the starting position.

Place the hands on the hips. Bend forward by creasing in the hips and maintaining a straight back and until the torso comes parallel to the ground. Slowly straighten up until you're back to the starting position.

The hip hinge is all about alignment and control. Don't rush your movements.

Reverse Snow Angels

Instead of lying flat on your back like you did as you make those snow angels during winter, you'll lie face down and flat on your belly. Do this on the carpet or use a mat for added comfort.

With the palm of your hands facing the ground, place the arms at the side of your torso while keeping the weight in the legs and hips evenly distributed.

Do not let your palms touch the ground. Slowly move the arms in an arching motion until your hands touch, keeping the arms straight the whole time. Yes, like making a snow angel. Slowly go back to the starting position, again without letting your arms touch the floor.

Locust

This is a more advanced weight-less back exercise, but this will activate all the muscles on your back. It was derived from a yoga position and will also work your legs and arms.

Start by lying down on your belly with the arms at the side and the legs straight. Rest your forehead on the floor and keep the palms up.

Slowly lift your head, chest, arms, and the legs and look at the ceiling. Balance on your abdominal area while raising the legs as high as you can.

Slowly go back to the starting position.

4 - The Biceps

The upper arm consists of the biceps and the triceps. Triceps are also worked when doing pushing exercises like pushups and dips. Developing or strengthening the bicep muscles without weights can be difficult but it can surely be done.

Let's look first at the anatomy of a bicep exercise. Basically, in order to develop your bicep muscles, you need to do a curling motion wherein you raise your lower arm towards your shoulders. This engages the bicep muscles but to keep it challenged, you need to incorporate some resistance.

Towel Curls

For this exercise, you'll need a bath towel. Roll it up lengthwise so it forms a thick rope then fold it in half. Sit on a chair then place a leg in the middle of the folded tower. Hold each end of the towel by gripping tightly with each hand.

Now slowly pull the ends of the towel up towards your shoulders without using your leg muscles. The weight of your leg then becomes the resistance for this exercise. The weight of the leg alone can prove to be a challenge for beginners and to add even more resistance, push away using your leg as you pull up the towel.

This exercise imitates doing barbell curls and is great for developing your biceps.

Arm Resistance Curls

So, you can't find a towel to do your bicep exercises? No problem. You can imitate a bicep concentration curl on one arm using the other arm as resistance. This routine is usually done by bodybuilders either as a contest pose or as a warm-up before they go on stage.

You can start by either sitting down on a chair or standing up. The arm being exercised should have its palm up and is placed at the side. Using the other arm, clasp your hands and slowly lift the arm on the side towards the shoulder. As you do this, push with the other arm to provide some resistance. The difficulty of this exercise can be varied by how much resistance you provide with the other arm.

Chin Up

OK. You might say I might be cheating because I'll be recommending an equipment for this exercise since it requires a pull-up bar. Well, you will still be using your body weight for this exercise. Also, you can buy a pull-up bar and put it on a door. It shouldn't cost you that much. This equipment is also versatile since you can do other exercises with it that can strengthen your back and abdominals.

Chin ups incorporate the curling motion as you pull yourself up and try to touch the bar with your chin. Start by gripping the bar firmly with your palms facing your body. The grip should also be shoulder width. Keeping your body straight, slowly pull your body up using your biceps and back muscles until your chin touches the bar. Slowly go back to the starting position.

This exercise is considered an advanced routine because you'll be lifting up your whole-body weight. You can begin with a bit of cheating by stepping on a chair and helping the pull-up motion by pushing down with your feet. Do this until you are able to do a chin up without the chair.

5 - The Triceps

Triceps actually compose a bigger part of your upper arms than biceps do. As the name implies, it's composed of three muscles and is generally used for pushing motion. You use the triceps when you do pushups, which also develop your chest muscles.

There are quite a number of triceps exercises you can do without using free weights but some of them will require equipment. These are routines you can do at home.

Narrow Pushup

Remember the narrow pushup in a previous chapter? That same exercise is actually also great for developing your triceps. Using a narrow grip when doing a pushup incorporates less of the chest muscles and more of the triceps muscles. This is a more difficult variation of the pushup since you'll be relying more on your triceps to push your body off the floor and triceps are generally weaker than chest muscles because they are smaller.

You can do some variations on the narrow pushup routing like putting one of the arms a bit farther away from the inner chests. This is great for challenging an arm or blasting through plateaus. You can also place a couple of thick books under one hand while doing the narrow grip pushup.

You can also do a diamond pushup. This is more difficult than a regular narrow pushup because the positioning of the hands will target your triceps muscles even more. With your index fingers and thumbs, you form a diamond and place it under your chest as you lie face down on the floor. Do the normal pushup motion. You'll feel more burn on your triceps using this variation. Remember to keep your back straight throughout the exercise.

The pushup is a versatile exercise since it can engage more than one muscle group. Variation and volume is the key.

6 - Legs

The muscles on your thighs form the biggest muscle group in your body. These muscles keep you upright when you are standing up and also helps move you around. Evolution did this, so you can walk, run, and jump.

Because a lot of movements are dependent on the legs, they are the easiest to challenge even without using free weights. Again, using free weights can help build bigger leg muscles but you don't need them if all you want is a great and challenging leg workout. Working the legs also engage the other muscles like the buttocks, the hamstrings, and the calves. It is important to wear knee sleeves that can provide the best support and compression.

These exercises will give you the best overall leg workout without the use of free weights.

Squats

The squat is the most common exercise for the legs. It's too common that most people tend to do it improperly. Some people even skip the squat since they say they do it almost every day when sitting down and standing up. But the foundation of all those lower-body workouts is the humble squat. Doing the squat routine can determine how you run, walk, lunge, or jump.

Start by standing with your feet shoulder width apart or wider. Lift your arms up to your front and hold them straight with your palms facing down. Some people would prefer crossing their arms over their shoulders. Holding your arms on the front helps you keep your balance while you do the squat.

Bend your legs on the knees slowly while keeping your back straight and looking straight in front of you. The feet should also lay flat on the floor throughout the exercise. Keep bending your legs until the thighs are parallel to the ground. Slowly stand up keeping the back straight until you're back to the starting position. That would be one repetition.

You might think it's too easy, but when you focus on doing squats for much more than ten repetitions, you'll find the real meaning of a leg day. The squat also works out your lower back, your buttocks, your hamstrings, and your calves.

For variety, you can widen your stance even more. By doing this, you'll engage a lot more of your inner leg muscles. Don't forget to keep your back straight and the width of your stance should be no more than what you are comfortable with or you'll risk injury.

Lunge

Lunges are the next best exercise for your legs, and again, they can effectively be done without using free weights. A lunge is actually a squat, but instead of using both legs, you'll only be using one while the other one stabilizes your pose.

Begin by standing with your legs a shoulder-width apart. Your arms should point down and at your sides. Using one leg, step back then both of your knees to form a 90-degree angle. Pause at this position so you can check if you have the proper form. The shin on the front leg should be vertical and the knee should not pass the toe. Be mindful of your posture by making sure that the torso is vertical and tall. Most people have a tendency to lean forward while doing the lunge. This will put extra strain on your back.

Using a slow, controlled motion, push with the leg on your front by driving your heel to the floor. Go back to the starting position and do the same motions with the other leg.

Glute Bridge

You've seen this move in countless exercise videos and although this exercise also effectively works out your buttocks, it also engages your upper leg muscles. The glute bridge is also recommended for those who cannot do a proper squat or lunge due to physical restraints.

Begin by lying down with your back flat on the floor. With your feet, a shoulder-width apart, bend your knees until they form a 90-degree angle. This will be your starting position.

Slowly push your heels down into the floor while raising your hips up. Do this until your torso is parallel to your thighs then squeeze your glutes and keep your abdomen tight to prevent arching. The shins should also be vertical. Slowly lower your back and go back to the starting position.

For variety, you can use a chair or a Swiss exercise ball to place your feet on. This will engage the thigh muscles and the glutes more.

Step Up

The step up is a very effective yet very low-risk exercise that you can do for your legs or the lower body in general. You can also incorporate this into your routine if you feel that one of your legs is weaker than the other.

You'll be needing a chair or a bench for this exercise. Start by placing a foot on the elevated platform and push down as you stand up straight. Make sure you are not hinging at your hips or leaning forward. Keep your body straight and vertical throughout the motion.

Single Leg Calf Raise

Your calves stabilize your legs as you walk, run, or simply stand up. It's one of the more worked out muscles in your body so growing or developing it can be challenging since it's used to daily torture. You can incorporate more resistance without using free weights by using only one leg.

Stand up straight and lift one of your legs up by bending on the knees. If you can't do this without wobbling, hold on to a chair or a door. Remember to use the least assistance as possible in maintaining your balance. Your goal is to challenge that calf.

Lift yourself up by pushing down with the ball of your foot until you can feel your calf tightening up. Go back to starting position. The idea here is to do the exercise until failure before you switch to the other foot.

7 - Conclusion

Having no free weights or specialized equipment should not be an excuse for not having a full body workout. You don't even have to go to the gym, spend money on gym memberships, or buy your own equipment. You can use your own body weight as resistance to tone or build muscles.

The idea here is variation and volume. You should vary your exercise routines to avoid plateaus. And since you'll be using your body weight for resistance, you should aim for volume. Most of the exercises here should be done until failure. That means until you can't do another repetition anymore. You can then take a minute or two of rest then begin again.

Happy exercising!

Thank You

As we reach the end of this book, I want to say thanks for reading this book.

I want to get this information out to as many people as possible. If you found this book helpful, I would greatly appreciate you leaving me a review. This helps others find the book as well.

This book was self-published with the amazing help of <u>Self-Publishing Made Easy Now!</u> [3] . You can grab a free copy of the checklist that started my journey here: <u>FREE Self-Publishing Checklist</u> [4] .

[3] https://selfpublishingmadeeasynow.com/xpjv

[4] https://selfpublishingmadeeasynow.com/free_checklist

Disclaimer

This document is geared towards providing exact and reliable information in regards to the topic and issue covered. The publication is sold on the idea that the publisher is not required to render an accounting, officially permitted, or otherwise, qualified services. If advice is necessary, legal, financial, medical or professional, a practiced individual in the profession should be ordered.

This information is not presented by a financial or medical practitioner and is for entertainment, educational and informational purposes only. The content is not intended as a substitute for professional medical advice, diagnosis, or treatment. Always seek the advice of your physician or other qualified health care provider with any questions you may have regarding a medical condition. Never disregard professional medical advice or delay in seeking it because of something you have read.

The information provided herein is stated to be truthful and consistent, in that any liability, in terms of inattention or otherwise, by any usage or abuse of any policies, processes, or directions contained within is the solitary and utter responsibility of the recipient reader. Under no circumstances will any legal responsibility or blame be held against the publisher for any reparation, damages, or monetary loss due to the information herein, either directly or indirectly.